COMBAT
KNEE PAIN
Naturally

IMPROVE KNEE FUNCTION TO CONQUER PAIN

DR. SUNIT S EKKA(PT)

COMBAT
KNEE PAIN
Naturally

IMPROVE KNEE FUNCTION TO CONQUER PAIN

PICTURE CREDITS

1. Knee Osteoarthritis: By BruceBlaus - Own work, CC BY-SA 4.0, **https://commons.wikimedia.org/w/index.php?curid=44968165**.
2. Hip abductors: By Beth ohara (Own work) CC-BY-SA-3.0 (http://creativecommons.org/licenses/by-sa/3.0/)], via Wikimedia Commons.
3. Hamstring muscle: BruceBlaus [CC BY-SA 4.0 https://creativecommons.org/licenses/by-sa/4.0)].
4. British Columbia Institute of Technology (BCIT). Download this book for free at http://open.bccampus.ca [CC BY 4.0 (https://creativecommons.org/licenses/by/4.0)]
5. Anatomy of knee: Servier Medical Art by Servier, https://smart.servier.com/

MESSAGE

Osteoarthritis knee is the major cause of knee pain and disability in the elderly. In a late OA case, the surgical replacement is the only way out.

Fortunately, you can minimize pain and disability with exercises and physiotherapy. Having said this, surgery can be avoided in the early stage of OA. Even in the late case, if you can't avoid it, exercises help it delay. Delaying surgery has its own benefit.

With this collection of the most effective exercises, I wish you all happy healing.

Dr Sunit Sanjay Ekka (PT)

BPT, SVNIRTAR.

Content

TREAT YOUR KNEE PAIN NATURALLY 1

HOW TO USE THIS BOOK? **ERROR! BOOKMARK NOT DEFINED.**

INTRODUCTION 11

WHAT IS OSTEOARTHRITIS KNEE? 14

ANATOMY OF KNEE JOINT 16

JOINT CHANGES IN OA KNEE 18

CLINICAL FEATURE OF OSTEOARTHRITIS KNEE PAIN 19

STAGES OF OA KNEE 21

EARLY STAGE OA KNEE 24

INTERMEDIATE STAGE 26

LATE STAGE 27

HOW TO MANAGE OA KNEE PAIN 29

KNEE REHABILITATION EXERCISES 32

KNEE JOINT MUSCLE ANATOMY 33

STRENGTHENING EXERCISES 36

1: STATIC QUADRICEPS EXERCISES 38

Description of static quadriceps exercises 39
The significance of static quadriceps exercises 40

2: DYNAMIC QUADRICEPS EXERCISES 43

Description of dynamic quadriceps exercises 44
The significance of exercise 45

3: ADDUCTOR STRENGTHENING EXERCISES 47

Description of adductor strengthening exercise 48

4: ABDUCTOR STRENGTHENING EXERCISES 52

Description of the exercise 53
The significance of the exercise 54

5: SHORT ABDUCTOR STRENGTHENING EXERCISES 57

Description of exercise 59
Significance of the exercise 60

6: KNEE FLEXOR STRENGTHENING EXERCISES 61

Description of exercise 62
The significance of the exercise. 63

7: CLOSED-LOOP QUADRICEPS STRENGTHENING EXERCISES 66

Description of exercise 67
The significance of the exercise 69

8: CALF MUSCLE STRENGTHENING EXERCISES 70

Description of exercise 70
Significance of exercise 72

STRETCHING EXERCISE 74

9: POSTERIOR KNEE CAPSULE STRETCHING EXERCISE 76

Description of the exercise 77
The significance of the exercise 78

PAIN MANAGEMENT TIPS 80

KNEE BRACES 81

Two types of knee brace are 81

LIFESTYLE MODIFICATION 83

EXERCISES 84

Recommended hydrotherapy exercises 84

CYCLING FOR KNEE PAIN 88

WHY SHOULD OSTEOARTHRITIS PATIENTS LOSE WEIGHT? 90

ACTIVITY RESTRICTION FOR OA KNEE SUFFERER 91

LATE STAGE OA KNEE 92

HOW EXERCISES CAN HELP AT THIS STAGE? 94

EXERCISES IN LATE STAGE 94

FINAL WORD 96

ABOUT THE AUTHOR 97

Forward

As an Occupational Therapist, I know Sunit Sanjay Ekka form since the last 16 years from now. He was my student at SVNIRTAR (Swami Vivekananda National Institute of Rehabilitation and Research).

I appreciate his dedication to his patient. His knowledge will guide you towards the proper direction of getting rehabilitation for your pain and disability.

Sunil Mokashi,
Ex-Head of the Department, Occupational Therapy.
SVNIRTAR (Govt of India)

Introduction

Osteoarthritis (OA) knee is the most common chronic disease and one of the leading causes of pain and disability worldwide. It affects the sufferer's ambulation, reduces the quality of life and social participation.

It mostly affects the aging population and is common after the age of 55 years. The prevalence of knee OA in men is lower compared with women. And females, particularly those equal to or more than 55 years of age, tended to have more severe OA in the knee. About 13% of women and 10% of men aged 60 years and older have symptomatic knee OA(Heidari).

In the early stage of OA knee, the sufferer complains of pain on stair climbing, getting up from crossed leg sitting. They will typically complain of pain in a particular position of knee when walking or standing. A crackling sound (medical term is crepitus) is a common symptom at this early stage.

As the degenerative process further precedes the knee pain becomes more apparent with daily activities. The sufferer will complain of difficulty in walking and climbing stairs due to severe knee pain. They will even have a struggle coming to standing from a chair or bed.

In a late case, the pain becomes so severe that it can make a person bed rid.

Depending on the severity of pain and disability, in this book, we will classify OA knee into three-stage. This will help you to understand your pain better and in turn, help to manage pain and exercise accordingly.

We will classify it into three stages:

1. Early stage.
2. Intermediate stage.
3. Late stage.

Though, your doctor is the best person to describe the stage of your OA knee, in the coming chapters we will cover all the stages in detail including sign and symptoms. This will help you to understand your knee pain.

Scientific studies have shown that the effectiveness of exercise is mostly seen in the first two stages, which is an early and intermediate stage. However, we will also cover the late stage and learn exercises and few effective tips that may help you.

Having said this, almost all exercises described in this book will be of most help to the early stage and intermediate stage.

The late stage is a very serious stage where there is a serious amount of irreversible damage in the articular surface amounting to make sufferer bed rid.

There are few exercises and pain-relieving tips that may help but in my experience knee replacement is the best option for late osteoarthritis knee sufferer.

However, exercises in this book can also help pre-operative preparations which are important for minimizing post-operative complications and better results of surgery.

With this I would like to wish all the osteoarthritis knee sufferer, happy healing and speedy recovery!

* * *

What is osteoarthritis knee?

Osteoarthritis (OA) knee is a painful knee condition that develops spontaneously with aging. It makes your knee look swollen and make daily activities like walking, stair climbing, squatting and, cross leg sitting a painful experience. In a severe case, one may even go bed rid.

To understand osteoarthritis, we first need to learn its terminology. The term osteoarthritis is actually a combination of two terms "*osteo*" and "*arthritis*".

Osteo means bone or related to bone and *arthritis* means inflammation of joints. In public health sectors, arthritis is a blanket term used to refer to more than 100 rheumatic diseases and conditions that affect the joints, the tissues surrounding the joints, and other connective tissue(Lespasio et al.).

When inflammation of knee joint (or any other joint) occurs due to the degenerative process of aging, weight, repeated microtrauma due to particular posture, resulting in wear and tear of the cartilage and underlying bone of knee is termed Osteoarthritis (OA) Knee.

So, how can we define OA knee?

Osteoarthritis knee is the degenerative joint disease that causes slow but irreversible damage to smooth cartilage of the knee joint, it becomes rough and eroded resulting in painful friction between the articular surfaces.

The knee articular joint surface is smooth because it is covered with smooth line of cartilage for a smooth and frictionless movement. In OA this surface becomes erode, this happens with increased wear and tear process on joint due to the affect of age, weight, and trauma to joint due to repetitive movements, in particular, squatting and kneeling(Heidari).

To understand this we need to learn a little about the anatomy of a normal knee joint.

Anatomy of knee joint

The knee joint is a movable hinge joint that allows a great degree of movement. The human body broadly consists of two types of joints, one is immovable and another is movable joint. As the name suggests, movable joints allow movement and its anatomy is different from an immovable joint.

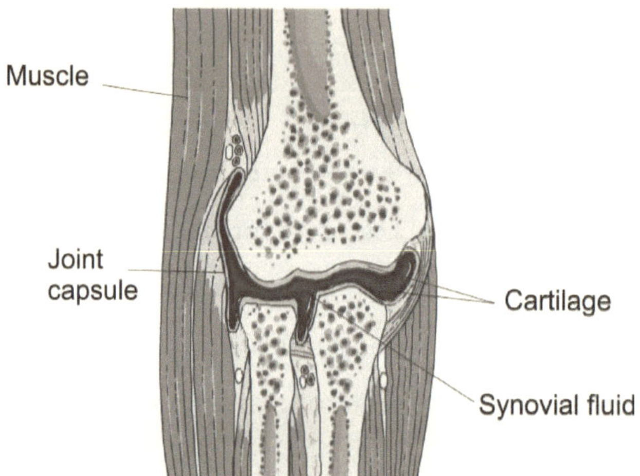

Figure 1: Anatomy of knee joint

The movable joint is surrounded by a capsule creating a joint space between the two articular surfaces. The joint space is filled with body fluid and has a very important role in acting like lubricants.

This lubricating body fluid is called synovial fluid and this is why the movable joints are also termed as a *synovial joint*. We can compare this fluid to lubricating fluid that we use in our bicycles and vehicles for smooth and frictionless movement of wheels.

The articular surface of a joint is the surface line that participates in the joint formation, and two articular surfaces make a joint.

In a normal joint, the two articular surfaces (surface of bone taking part in joint formation) are smooth because it is laminated with cartilage. Smooth enough to allow frictionless, pain-free movement of joint. Just beneath cartilage is subchondral bone.

So, what actually goes wrong in osteoarthritis?

Joint changes in OA knee

In osteoarthritis, this articular surface becomes eroded and rough. You can see the illustration of a normal joint and an osteoarthritic joint.

When a person suffering from OA knee walks, the rough surface comes in contact and produces friction. And yes, this friction makes the joint movement painful.

As a result, swelling develops around it and if not addressed properly, the continuous friction further degenerates the joint.

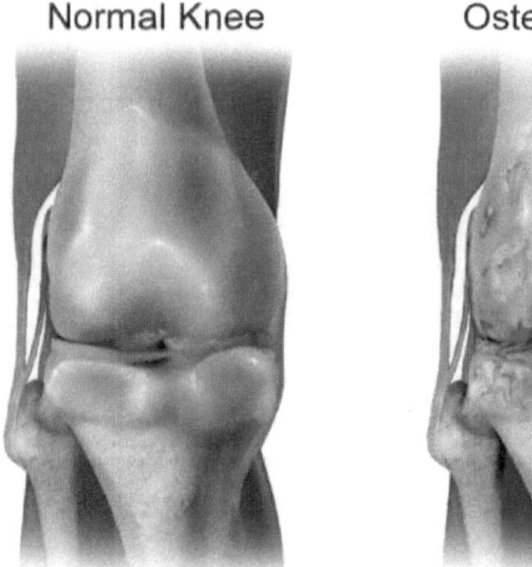

Figure 2: Normal vs OA knee

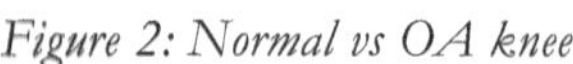

Clinical feature of osteoarthritis knee pain

In my 11 years of physiotherapy career, I have seen many OA knee cases. The most common complaint they report is knee pain during walking and stair climbing.

If they sit on the floor, it becomes a struggle to get up and even coming to a standing position from sitting on the bed is painful.

Pain and stiffness in the morning, after sitting, or after prolonged rest are most common. Over time, painful symptoms may occur more frequently, including during rest or at night(Lespasio et al.).

Let's discuss the symptoms one by one.

1. **Insidious onset of pain with activities involving weight-bearing over the knee:** Weight-bearing activities such as walking, stair climbing, squatting (eg. Using Indian mode of the toilet), crossed leg sitting.

2. **Morning pain and stiffness:** The patient will complain of knee pain and stiffness in the morning. This may subside with movement and

as the day progress.

3. **Crepitus:** Crepitus is a crackling sound that comes out of joint when the joint is in motion. This is very common with OA knee. The patient often complains of the crackling sound from the knee during the knee movement.

4. Boney enlargement and articular destruction are seen in the X-Ray.

* * *

Stages of OA knee

As we have discussed in our introduction that the osteoarthritis is a degenerative disease and depending on the severity of degeneration of OA knee we can classify it in stages. Starting from the early stage through intermediate stage to late stage the degeneration becomes more serious and irreversible in nature.

Doctors use X-ray radiological investigation to assess these changes. The joint erosion can be detected in an X-ray film. Based on these radiological findings Kellgren and Bier in 1957 first graded the severity of OA(KELLGREN and LAWRENCE).

In this chapter, we will take this gradation into account and will try to study it under the early stage, intermediate stage and late stage.

As in earlier surveys (Kellgren and Lawrence, 1952; Lawrence, 1955), osteoarthrosis was divided into five grades as follows(Kohn et al.):

- None (0)
- Doubtful (1)
- Minimal (2)
- Moderate (3)
- Severe (4)

Grade 0 thus indicated a definite absence of x-ray changes of OA, so let's ignore this grade. Grade 1 and Grade 2 OA in our opinion definitely present though of minimal severity, so let us place these two grades under the *early stage* of our classification.

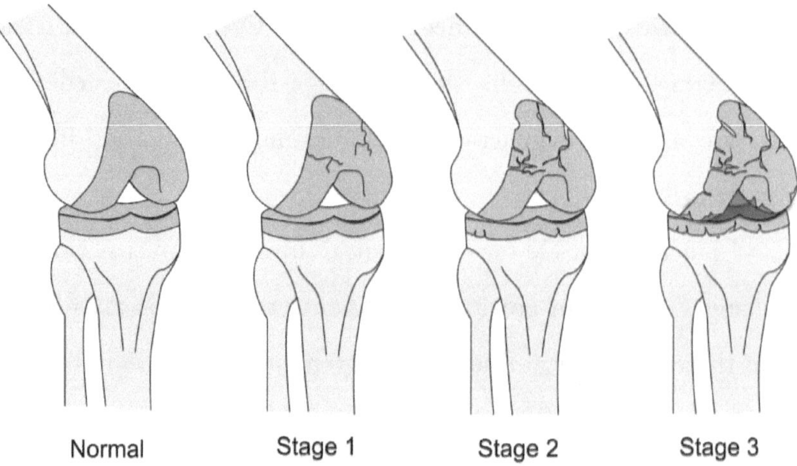

Figure 3: Stages of OA knee

Likewise let's place Grade 3 under *mid stage* and Grade 4 under *late stage*.

In the coming chapter, we will try to understand the degenerative changes that are seen during these grades and how it is manifested by signs and symptoms.

So, let us begin our discussion with early stage OA knee.

Early stage OA knee

The early stage is the starting stage of OA knee when a person first complains of mild knee pain. There is an increasing awareness on the importance in identifying early phases of the degenerative processes in knee osteoarthritis (OA), the period of the disease when there might still be some regenerative ability of the articular cartilage, which is permanently lost in the advanced disease stages.

The person appreciates pain only in a particular position of leg and foot in standing or stair climbing.

Pain is so mild that often sufferer ignores it by relating it to daily activities.

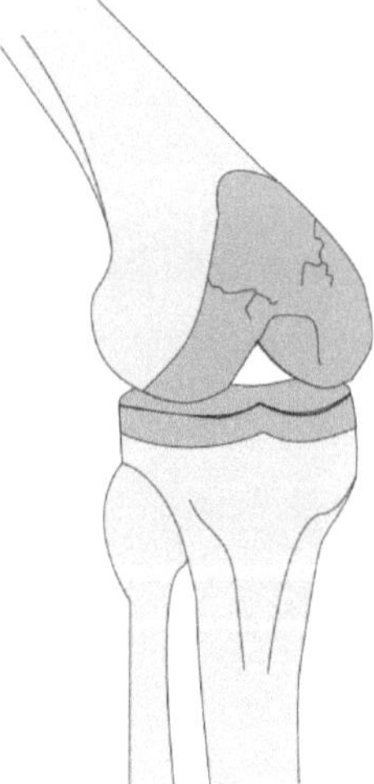

Figure 4: Early stage OA knee

As we had placed the Kellgren–Lawrence (KL) Grade 1 and 2 under this stage, let us learn what changes inside our knee joint occurs during this stage of OA knee.

- There is a doubtful narrowing of joint space narrowing.
- Possible osteophytes.

Normally there is optimal space between the joints and as we have already studied, it is filled with synovial fluid. In OA knee, this joint space tends to decrease and in this stage, it appears to have started to decrease but still it is doubtful.

Also, the X-Ray study reveals that osteophytes formation starts to appear on the joint line. These are small bony projections that limit the joint motion and produces pain on moving the joint.

Intermediate stage

Intermediate stage is mid way between the early stage and late stage. We can study the characteristic of this stage as Grade 3 of kellgren Lawrence system.

Grade III Kellgren Lawrence is characterized by

1. Multiple osteophytes,

2. Definite joint space narrowing,

3. Sclerosis [seen as increased white areas in the bone at the joint margin] and

4. Possible bony deformity.

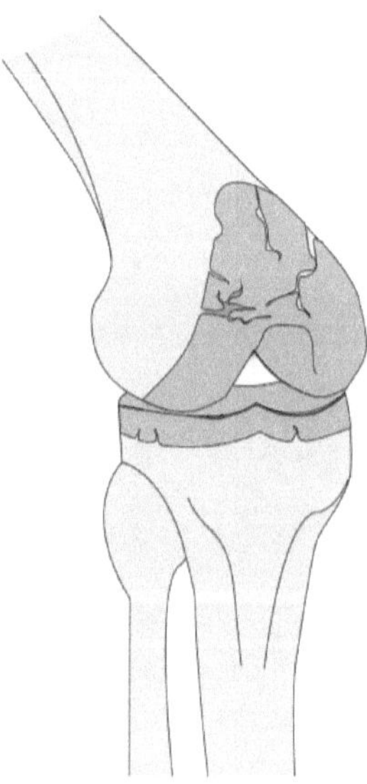

Figure 5: Intermediate stage

As the wear and tear process further degenerates the early stage OA knee, it reaches the intermediate stage. In this stage the joint space further reduces and becomes more oblivious. The extra bone formation or osteophytes formation on the lips of joint limits the joint movement due to pain and stiffness.

Late stage

Most painful and severe stage, there's considerable loss of joint space. Joint space becomes so narrow that even the articular surface comes in contact with each other.

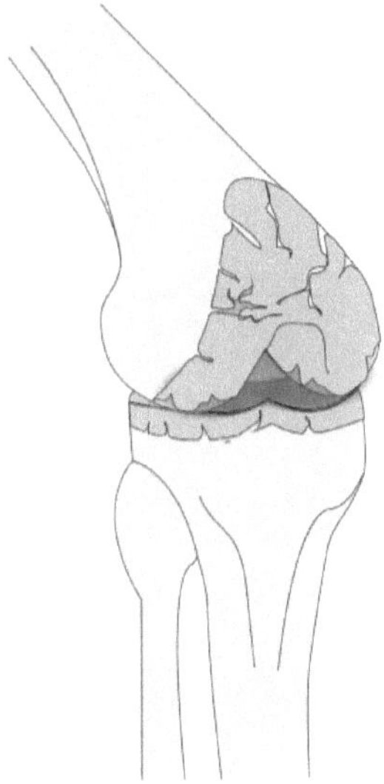

Figure 6: Late stage

The cartilage is almost gone and the smooth articular surface becomes rough.

It is characterized by

1. large osteophytes,

2. Marked joint space narrowing,

3. Severe sclerosis, and

4. Definitely bony deformity.

Late stage OA pain may lead to anxiety, depression, fear of movement, and poor psychological outlook. The fear of movement may prevent participation in exercise and social events which could lead to further physical and social isolation (Kevin R. Vincent, 2012).

* * *

How to manage OA knee pain

There is no cure for osteoarthritis knee and typically a person lives approximately 30 years of life with this disease. However, we can manage it and prevent early stage proceeding to become intermediate or late stage. If not prevent, at least we can delay the process of degradation.

Most of the medical treatment is symptomatic that results in short-term palliation of symptoms with little consideration of long-term risk. Ironically, patients with OA knee, Physical Therapy and lifestyle counseling seem underutilized while pain medication use is increased(Khoja et al.).

There is enough research to prove the effectiveness of lifestyle interventions such as weight loss and exercise, these should be advocated in all patients due to the low risk of harm. The use of

NSAIDs should be minimized to avoid gastrointestinal complications(Charlesworth et al.).

In this book, we will cover the management of osteoarthritis knee under headings:

1. Knee rehabilitation exercises.
2. Pain management tips.
3. Lifestyle modification.

In the following chapters, we will give more concentration on the knee rehabilitation exercises; along with it we will also consider lifestyle modifications which are important for overall effectiveness of exercise. I have picked the exercises that I usually prescribe to my patient at our physiotherapy center and I have practically experienced its positive result. We will learn each individual exercise thoroughly, covering topics such as its affects, anatomy and its significance.

In addition to this, we will also discuss some of the most effective conservative tips to get rid of pain symptoms.

Please note that the pain-relieving tips will give you temporary relief, for a long term affect one needs to focus on exercises and lifestyle modifications. However, pain relief will encourage you to continue with the exercises. After all, no one likes to perform exercises in pain, isn't it?

This also points us to a very important fact that not all exercises are beneficial in different stages of OA knee. In fact, most of the exercises are very difficult to carry out in the late stage and it may even aggravate the symptoms.

For this matter, I have structured this book such that we will first cover all the basic exercises. In a later chapter, we will learn which exercises are to be performed in which stage and how we can add slight variation (like the addition of weight) to serve that particular stage.

Let's start with knee rehabilitation exercises.

* * *

Knee rehabilitation exercises

For the long term management of OA knee, conservative management is the preferred mode of treatment. However, conservative treatment is advocated in patients with early to intermediate stage OA of the knee, late stage may require surgical intervention. But research also backs the fact that exercises in late stage may help to delay the surgery, and it is performed as a pre-operative treatment regimen.

Due to knee pain, the physical activities of the sufferer decline that result in secondary muscular weakness around the knee. Research has also revealed that muscle weakness (quadriceps muscle in particular) can become one of the reasons for osteoarthritis knee(Slemenda et al.), forming a vicious cycle of quadriceps weakness and OA knee pain.

Because muscle weakness is associated with pain and physical dysfunction and influences the progression of the disease(Slemenda et al.) in patients with OA of the knee, muscle strengthening is a key component in cases of OA.

However, knee rehabilitation exercises also include a few stretching exercises. And the good thing is that all of these exercises can be performed at home. I have practically experienced with my patient that a simple program of home quadriceps exercises can significantly improve self-reported knee pain and function(O'Reilly et al.).

It would be wise to cover some of the anatomical basics of muscle around the knee joint for a better and clear picture of role of exercises in this kind of pain.

Knee joint muscle anatomy

Our knee joint motion is controlled by various muscle and muscle group surrounding the knee and the thigh. The actions of these muscles bring about motion of bending and extending knee.

These muscles or muscle group are located all around our thigh. Look at your thigh, observe its bulkiness, it is due to the bulkiness of muscles. They are present on the front, back, and sides of thigh as you can see in the figure below.

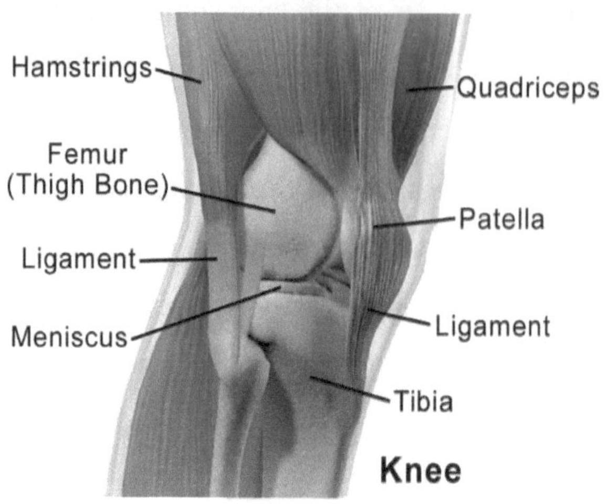

Figure 7

These muscles are

1.   Front: Quadriceps muscle.

2.   Inner side: Adductor group of muscle.

3.   Outer side: Abductor group of muscle.

4.   Behind: knee flexor group of muscles.

Every muscle or muscle group has a very specific role and together, in a well-coordinated manner, they bring the motion in the knee joint.

Quadriceps muscle in the front of thigh is responsible for knee extension (straightening) motion. The opposite action i.e. bending of knee is due to the action of muscle on back of thigh (hamstring).

The function of adductor muscle (on inner side of thigh) and abductor muscle group is to move our leg towards body and away from the body respectively. Although, there action does not cause any motion in knee joint but they do have very important role in knee biomechanics.

In OA knee, these muscles become weak due to long-term immobility or decreased mobility; decreased mobility is due to pain and disability. A weak muscle is incapable of holding the joint which resulting to alter the normal biomechanics and increased loading over the articular cartilage.

Therefore, it is essential to strengthening the muscle of knee joint by strengthening exercises. In coming chapter we will cover the details of all these muscle anatomy and how we can strengthen it individually.

* * *

Strengthening exercises

A strong muscle around the knee acts as strong pillars and they prevent the articular cartilage from coming in contact with each other. In OA knee, muscle strengthening exercises helps restoring normal knee biomechanics, resulting in a decreased joint loading rate or localized stress in the articular cartilage.

A strong muscle thereby plays an important role in delaying initiation and ameliorating the progression of knee OA(Fransen et al.).

Muscle strengthening exercise is also known as muscle resistance exercises. Muscle strengthening through resistance exercise (RX) increases physical function, decreases pain due to OA, and reduces self-reported disability (Kevin R. Vincent, 2012).

Components of a strengthening program include

1. Resistance load,
2. Repetitions,
3. Velocity of movement and
4. Frequency of sessions per week.

A periodic increase in the resistance load for each exercise permits continued muscular adaptations over time. Resistance can be applied through various methods.

- Body weight: in our case it's the weight of leg.
- Resistance bands: such as Theraband.
- Free weights: we will use weight cuff.
- Machines.

All the exercises we are going to discuss will follow a common regimen that involves exercise three days per week, with 2–3 sets per exercise at 8–15 repetitions per set.

With this, let us jump start our actual exercises.

1: Static Quadriceps Exercises

Starting position

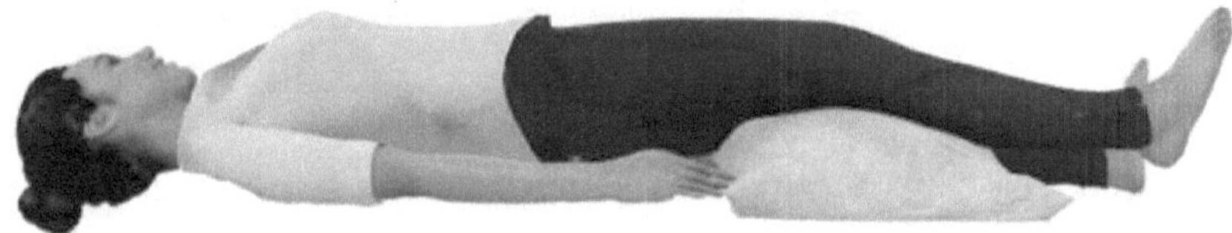

Figure 8

Target position

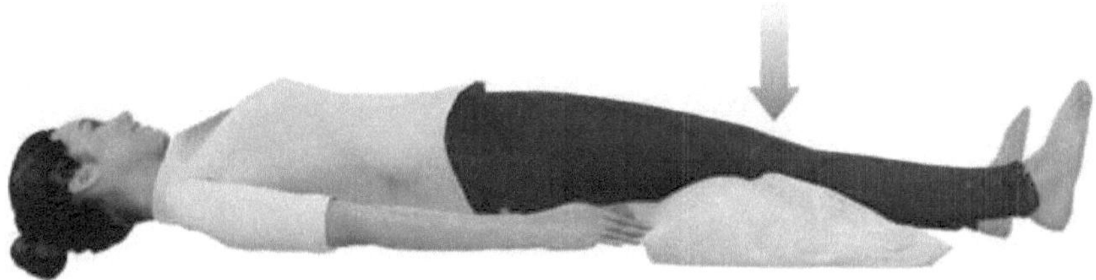

Figure 9

Description of static quadriceps exercises

This exercise is also known as knee press exercise. It is called a static exercise because there is no joint motion while performing exercise but still there's a considerable amount of muscle contraction.

This exercise is especially important when one is suffering from very severe knee pain. However, this is the most important exercise of all which is commonly prescribed worldwide by physician, surgeon and physical therapist alike.

The best thing about this exercise fits into all the three stage of OA and easy to learn and perform. So, before we learn its significance of this exercise and the muscle group it benefits, let's learn its technique.

Technique

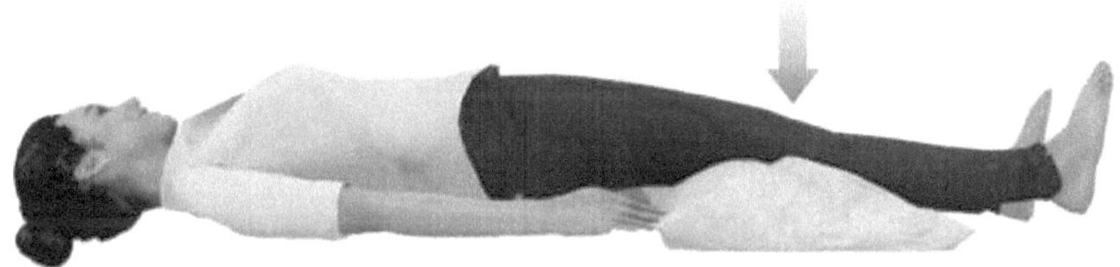

Figure 10

1.   Lie down flat on your back as shown in the figure.

2.   Put a pillow (or bed sheet roll/towel roll) below the knee.

3.   Press the pillow and hold it in the pressed position for 5 seconds (count 5) and then release it.

4.   Repeat this exercise for a minimum of 30 times in a single session, thrice daily

5.   As pain reduces it can be repeated to as many times as tolerated.

The significance of static quadriceps exercises

This exercise is to strengthen the quadriceps muscle. It is the biggest muscle in the body, a group of four muscles present on the front of our thigh. This is why it is termed as quadriceps i.e. *quad= four, ceps=muscles.* Look at your bulky muscle on the front of the thigh, they are the quadriceps muscle.

All four muscles arise from the different regions over ilium (front part of hip bone) and merge together to form quadriceps tendon and insert to the upper part of the knee cap (patella bone).

The figure below illustrates the quadriceps muscle and its two parts, the vastus lateralis and rectus femoris.

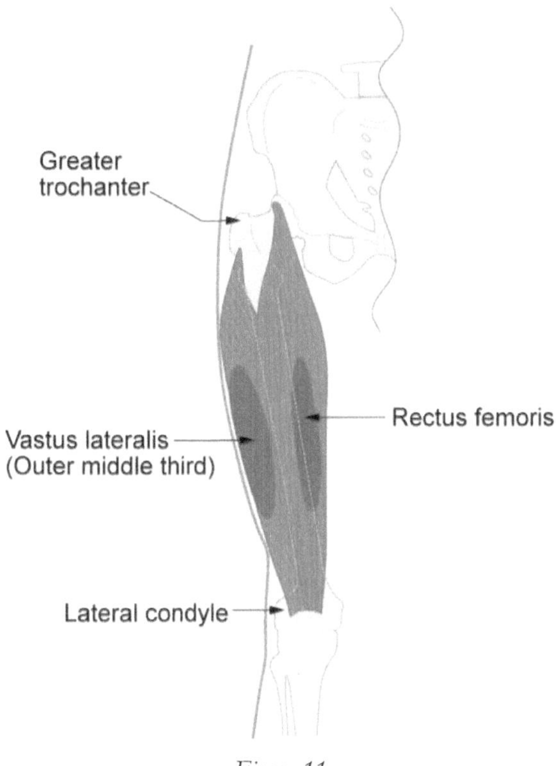

Figure 11

It has a very important function in extending the knee joint, that is when this muscle comes into action it brings straightening motion in the knee joint.

In persons with symptomatic osteoarthritis of the knee, quadriceps muscle weakness is common and is widely believed to result from disuse atrophy secondary to joint pain(Slemenda et al.).

Bullet points

1. This exercise helps in strengthening of the quadriceps muscle. Quadriceps muscle lies in the front of the thigh.
2. The function of this muscle is to extend the knee joint.

3.   The special thing about this exercise is, it is done
     without any movement of the joint. This is why it is
     called "static".

* * *

2: Dynamic Quadriceps Exercises

Contrary to the above quadriceps exercise, this exercise involves movement of limb and this is why it is called as dynamic exercise. The other term of this exercise is straight leg raise exercise.

Starting position

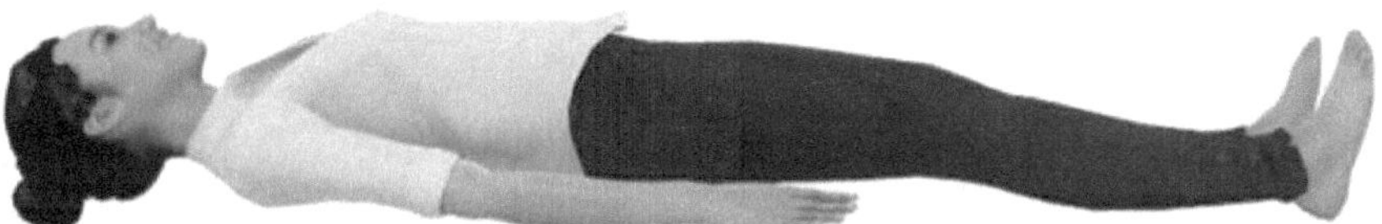

Figure 12

Target posture

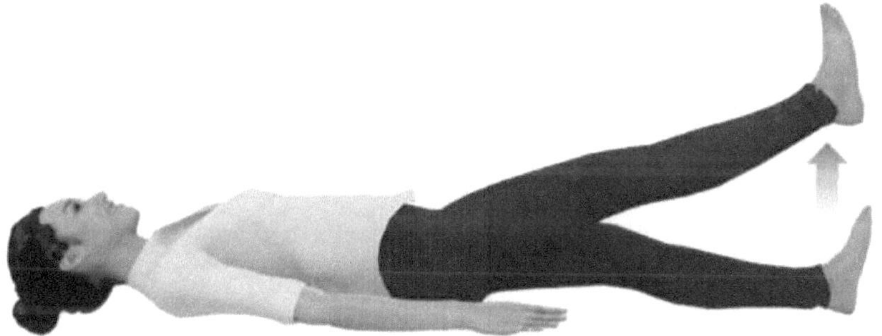

Figure 13

Description of dynamic quadriceps exercises

This exercise is also termed straight leg raise, in which one has to raise the leg maintaining knee joint in a straight position. Observe that contrary to the above exercises, in this exercise there is motion in the hip joint. This is why it is called as dynamic quadriceps exercise.

Also, note that here the weight of the leg is acting as resistance. As we progress with this exercise, we can add weight starting with half a kilogram of weight to make it more resistive. And further progression is made by adding an additional 0.5 kg till we reach to a total of 2 kg of weight.

We recommend adding of weight by using a weight cuff strapped just above the ankle joint. If you don't have weight cuff at home, you may use a 1 kg salt packet and use towel to wrap it around lower leg.

It would be wise if exercise is done on both the legs alternately. Below is the exact technique of performing this exercise.

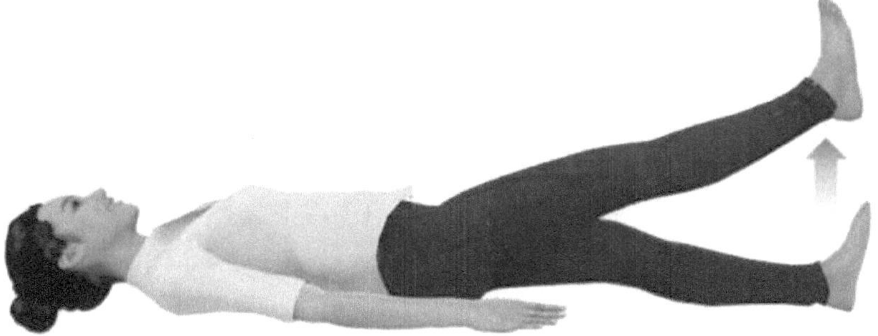

Figure 14

1. Your starting position should be lying straight on your back and hands by the side.

2. Now, slowly lift your leg keeping the knee straight.

3. Lift it to no more than 30 degrees of angle

4. Hold it for 5 seconds and then lower it down slowly.

5. Repeat step 2,3 and 4 on the opposite leg.

6. Repeat it for a minimum of 10 times in a single session.

7. Use weight cuff starting with 0.5 kg weight and progress to 1 kg, through 1.5 kg to 2 kg of weight.

The significance of exercise

This exercise is also used the strengthen the quadriceps muscle, however, it is more resistive than the static quadriceps exercise. This is because the person is lifting the weight of leg against the gravity and quadriceps muscle is working more the perform this action.

Bullet points:

1. The difference between the static quadriceps and dynamic quadriceps exercise is, the dynamic exercise involves movement of lower limb at the hip joint.
2. Note that the leg is being raised and lowered.
3. It is more resistive in nature than the static quadriceps exercise.

* * *

3: Adductor Strengthening Exercises

This strengthening exercise is to strengthen the muscle of the inner side of the thighs. The medical term for this muscle group is the adductor group of muscle. Before we dig deep, the figure below illustrates the exercise procedure.

Starting posture

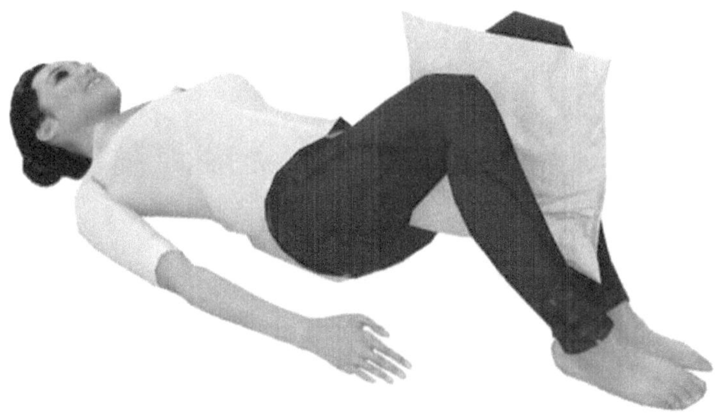

Figure 15

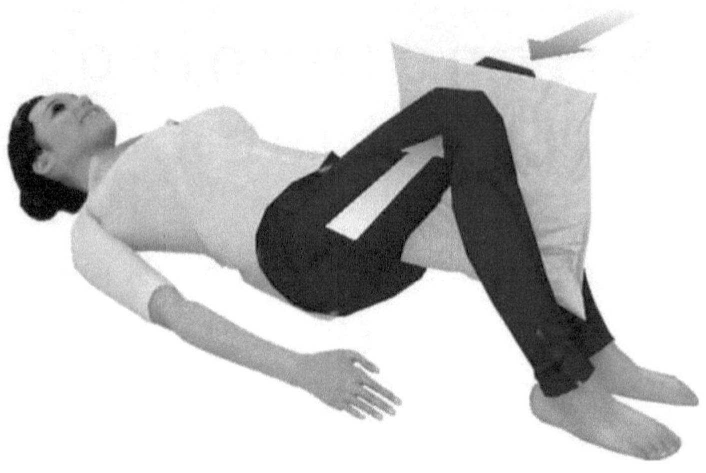

Figure 16

Description of adductor strengthening exercise

This is a very simple, effective exercise yet often ignored by many rehabilitation professionals. Look at the illustration, in which a pillow is kept between the thighs. The arrow mark signifies that it is pressed or to be specific, compressed between the thighs.

Often a single pillow isn't sufficient to bring enough resistance, in which case you may fold the pillow or you may use two pillow as per your convenience.

So, what's the exact technique?

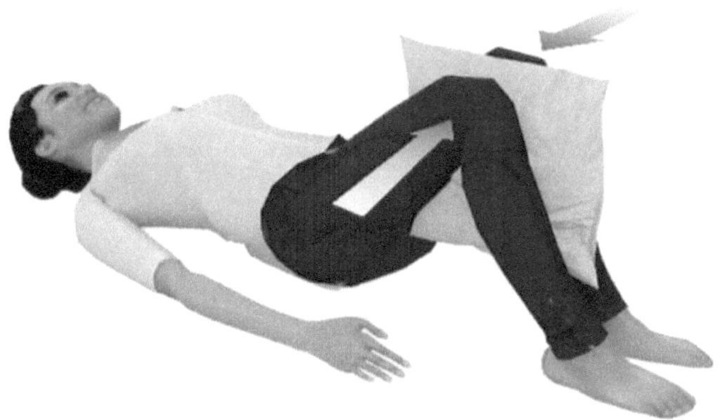

1. Lie down flat on your back keeping the knee in the bend position. Hands are kept by the side of body.

2. Keep a firm pillow between the thighs. Pillow should be thick enough to allow sufficient press, if not then make the pillow fold at the center. You may use two pillows altogether.

3. Press the pillow between the thighs, hold it for 5 seconds and then release it slowly. The best way is to count 1 to 5 for holding it for 5 seconds duration.

4. Repeat this for a minimum of 30 to 40 times in a single session.

The significance of the exercise

This exercise is meant to strengthen the hip adductor muscles.

Though its action has not effect on motion of knee joint, it does have a great influence on the biomechanics of the knee joint.

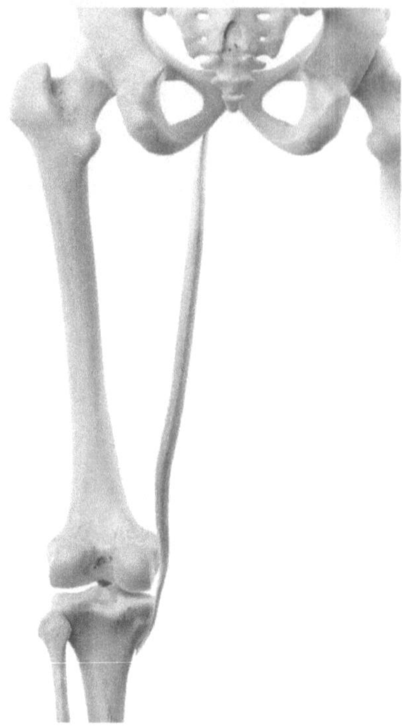

They are present on the inner side of the thigh and has important function to bring the adduction movement at the hip joint.

Adduction movement is a movement of body part towards the body, this is why it is termed as a hip adductor group of muscles. They are a group of five muscles.

Bullet points:

1. Adductor muscles lie on the inner side of the thigh.

2. It has a very important function of moving the leg towards the body.

3. Placing a pillow between the knee and pressing it results in motion of thigh inwards. Thus, this exercise is used to strengthen the adductor muscle of the thigh.

*　*　*

4: Abductor strengthening exercises

As the name suggests, abductor strengthening exercise is to strengthen muscle opposite to the above-discussed adductor muscle.

They are abductor group of muscle; let's start with these two illustrations showing the starting and target position of the exercise.

Starting posture

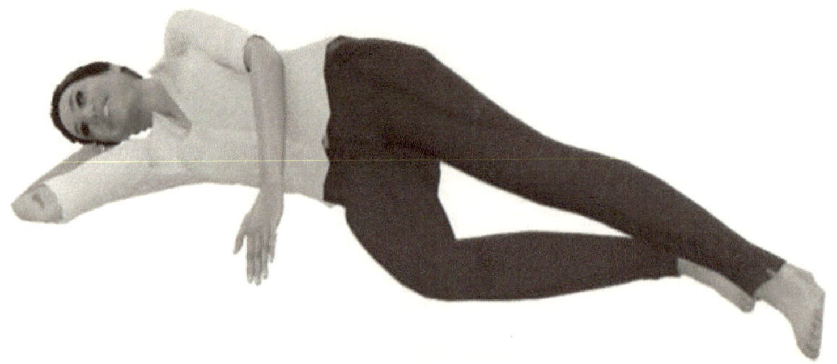

Figure 17

Target posture

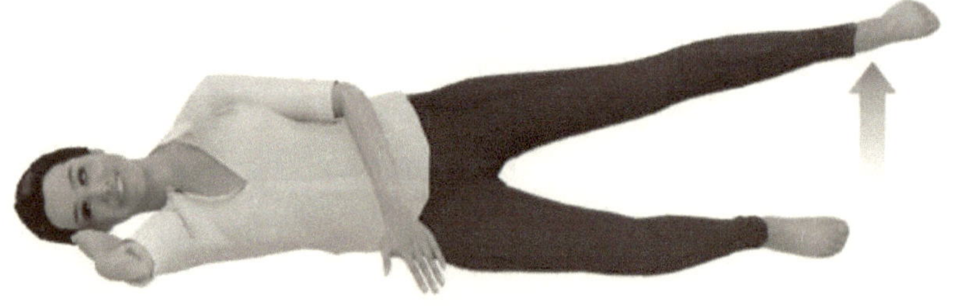

Figure 18

This is also a kind of *straight leg raise* exercise; the only difference is it is performed in a side-lying position. The leg on which the exercise is performed is kept on the top.

Having said this, let's suppose you want to exercise the left knee; place the left leg on top by side-lying on the right side (as in the figure below).

Let's dig deeper into its technique.

Technique

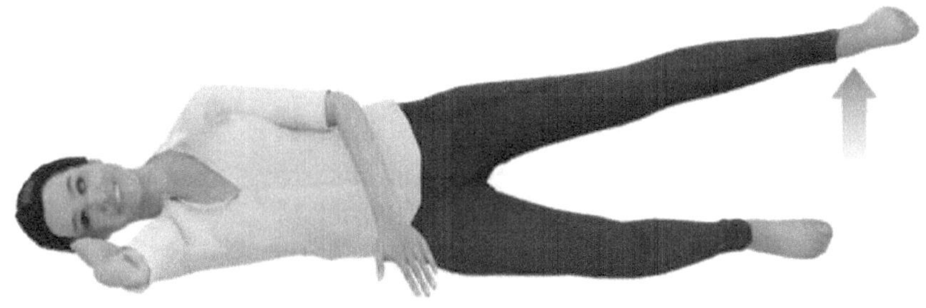

Figure 19

1. Lie down on your side (left or right).
2. As a rule of thumb, the knee which has to be exercised should be kept on top.

3. The knee which lies below is kept in bending position; this is to give a wide base of support and good stabilization.

4. For example, if you have to perform the exercise on the right knee, lie down on your left side while keeping the left knee slightly bent.

5. Now, slowly raise the right leg to not more than 30 degrees of angle.

6. Hold it for 5 seconds and lower it down slowly.

7. Repeat it for a minimum of 10 times in a single repetition.

The significance of the exercise

This is an abductor strengthening exercise and its purpose is to strengthen the hip abductors group of muscles.

They are the opposite of what we just discussed above, the adductor muscles. They are muscles of the outer/ adductor compartment of the thigh and are present on the outer side of the thigh.

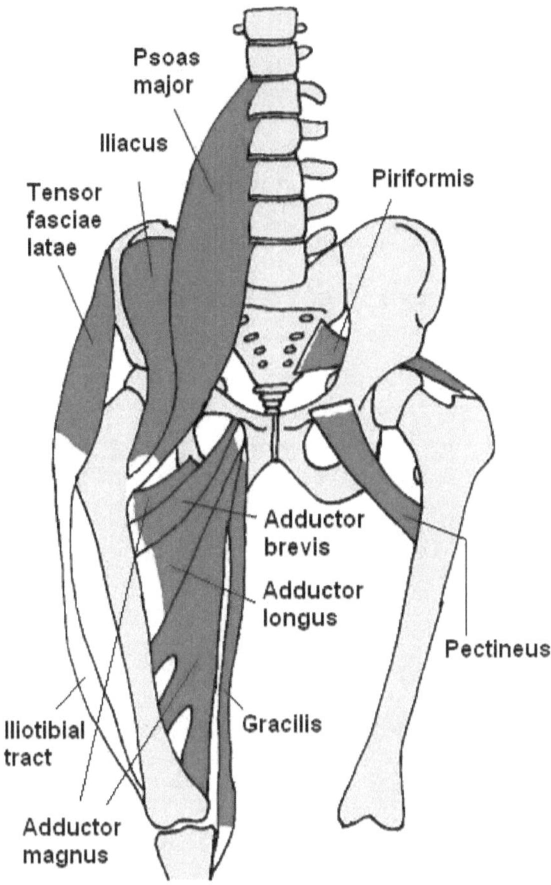

Figure 20: Three abductors

The action of these muscles produces the abduction movement of the thigh. Abduction means the thigh and leg move away from the body. The strong abductor muscle is also important for normal biomechanics of the knee joint.

Bullet points:

1. Abductor's muscle is opposite to the adductor muscle.

2.   They are situated on the outer side of the knee. Obviously, its function is to move the leg towards outside.

3.   Additional weight using weight cuff is used to increase the resistance load periodically. Proceed by adding 0.5 kg weight through 1 kg, 1.5 kg up to 2 kg of load.

∗ ∗ ∗

5: Short abductor strengthening exercises

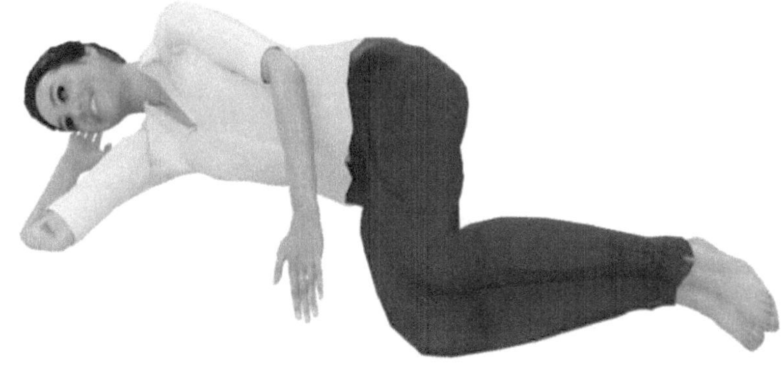

Figure 21

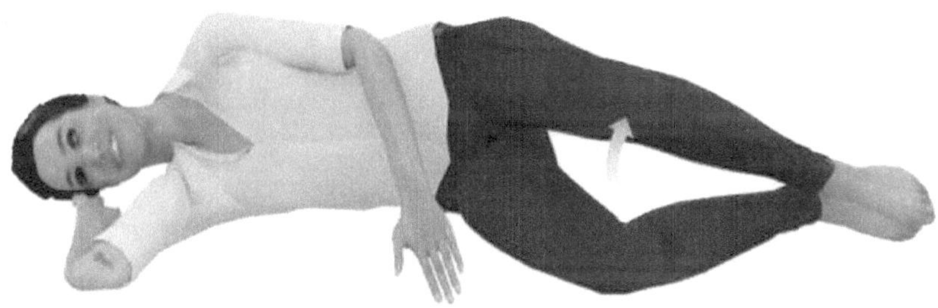

Figure 22

The 5th exercise is short abductor exercise and is for strengthening the short abductor muscle. They have same action is as abductor with a variation on hip position. The technique is also almost same as above with slight modification as in the illustration below

The starting position of the exercise is almost the same as the previous exercise; the only difference is the top lying leg should also be kept in bending position.

Another difference is, unlike in long abductor strengthening exercise, here there's no *straight leg raise* process. You just need to raise the knee keeping the foot in contact with each other.

Here's the step-by-step procedure.

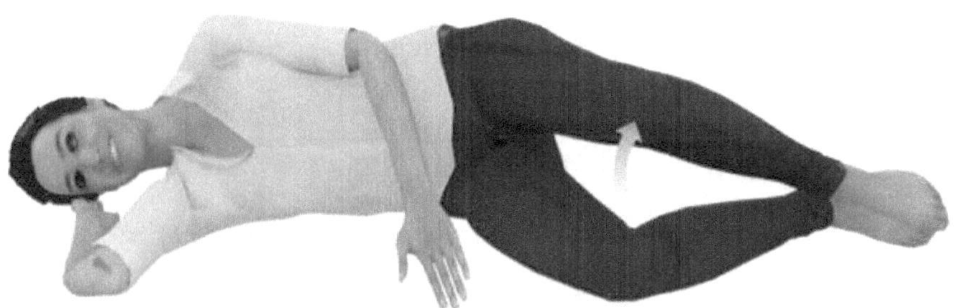

Figure 23

Technique

1. Lie down on your side (left/ right), the leg on which the exercise has to be performed is kept on top.

2. Keep both the knee in the bending position as shown in the figure.

3. Slowly raise the knee on the top while making sure that the foot is still kept in contact with each other.

4. Repeat it for a minimum of 30 to 40 times in a single session.

Significance of the exercise

Both long and short abductors are present on the outer side of the thigh, but they slightly differ in their actions.

Short abductor produces hip abduction movement in a position of hip flexion and slight knee flexion. Its action also influences the biomechanics of the knee joint.

Bullet points:

1. Like long abductors, short abductor **muscle is** also present on the outer side of the thigh and has the same function as the long ones.

2. Actually, this muscle group comes in action when hip joint is flexed midway. In this hip position, it is the main abductor of hip joint.

* * *

6: Knee flexor strengthening exercises

On the back of thigh is present hamstring muscle and its contraction produces knee flexion motion. This is the reason it is called as knee flexor and we are going to learn its strengthening exercise. The figure below is an overview of this exercise.

Starting posture

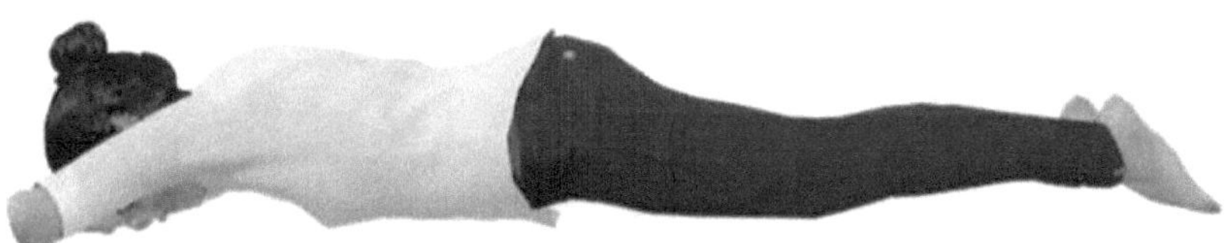

Figure 24

Target posture

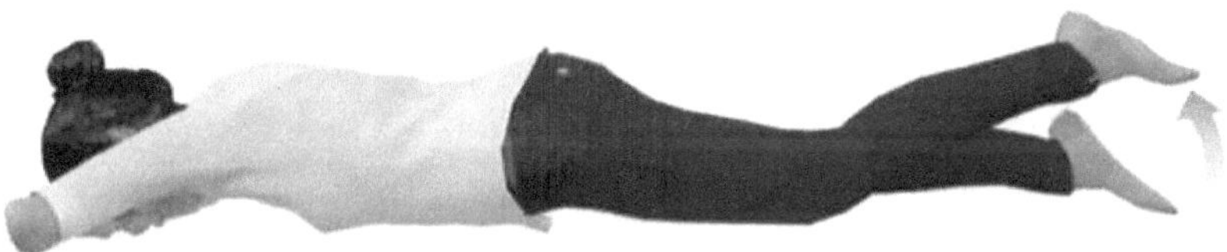

Figure 25

D e s c r i p t i o n   o f   e x e r c i s e

As you have seen in the illustration above, it is performed in the prone lying position, lying on the tummy is termed a prone lying. You may use a pillow for the head as per convenient.

As usual, try to maintain knee in the fully extended position. I would like to again mention that it is also a kind of *straight leg raise* but in a prone position.

Here is its exact technique.

T e c h n i q u e

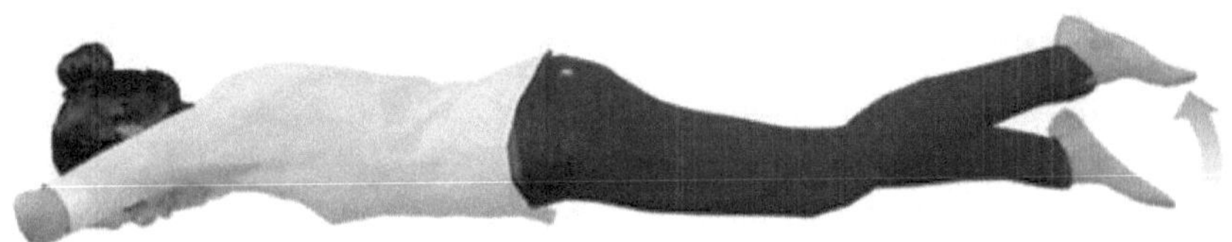

Figure 26

1. Start it by Lying down straight on your tummy (prone lying).
2. Slowly raise your leg as shown in the figure to not more than 30 degrees of angle. Knee should be maintained in straight position.
3. Hold it for 5 seconds and then lower it down slowly.

4.   Repeat the above process alternately on opposite leg.

5.   You should give at least 10 repetitions in a single session.

The Significance of exercise.

This group of muscles is present on the flexor compartment of the thigh which is situated on the back of our thigh. They are also called as hamstring muscle.

Hamstring muscles are bulky and very strong muscles formed by a grouping of three muscles. The muscles are the semimembranosus, semitendinosus, and biceps femoris muscles.

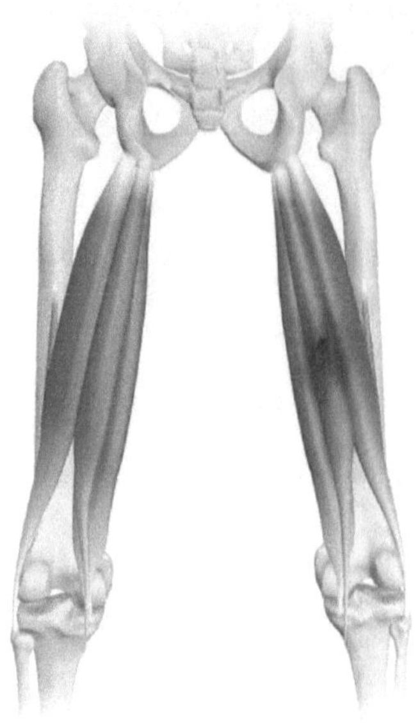

Figure 27: Hanstring muscle

Its action is very important for knee flexion and hip extension motion. Palpate your back of the thigh to feel its bulkiness.

Bullet points:

1. In the above chapters, we discussed muscle which functions to:　　　Extend the knee (Quadriceps), Move leg inwards (Adductors), Move the leg outwards (Abductors).

2. Now, the only muscle we are left with is the muscle that brings a bending motion of the knee called knee flexors.

3. So this exercise helps to strengthen the muscle on the backside of the knee.

* * *

7: Closed-loop quadriceps strengthening

These are land based exercise and are as simple as it sounds complicated. This illustration gives a clear picture of the exercises and note that it is performed in standing position on land/ floor.

Starting posture and Target posture

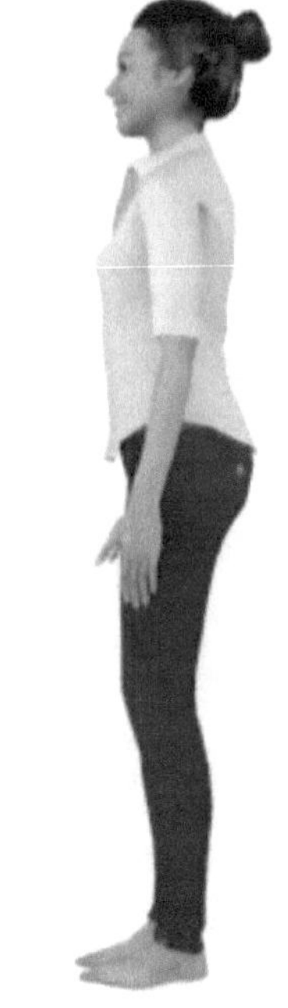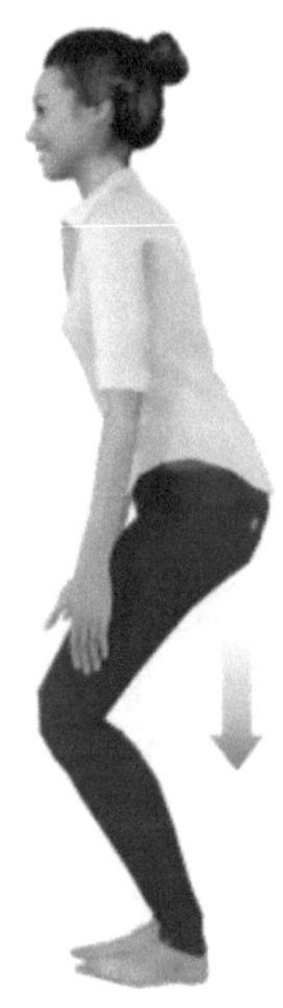

Figure 28

It is also known as the semi-squat position and we have to bend at our knee hip half way of squatting.

This exercise is called closed-loop exercise because, when doing half squatting, these movements happen in a loop:

1. Forward bending at the lower back.

2. Forward bending at both the hip joint.

3. Bending of both the knee.

4. Bending movement at both the ankle.

It is a land-based exercise and the technique of exercise is very simple, let's find out how to do closed-loop exercise.

Technique

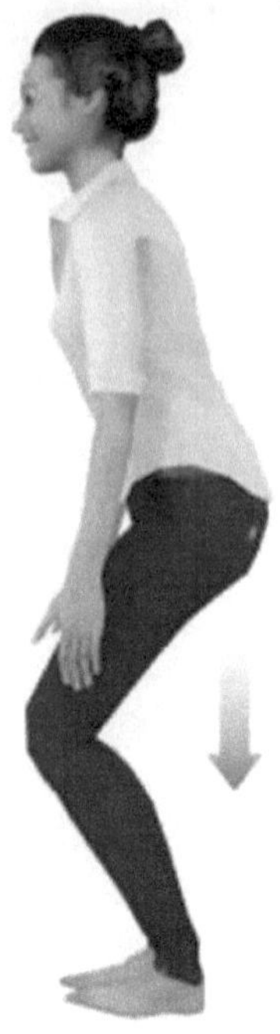

Figure 29

1. Stand straight with the feet kept apart.

2. Now, bend on your knees as shown in the figure, note that bending is halfway of the full squatting position. Then come back to the standing position slowly and steadily.

3. If it is difficult for you, then you may lean your back to the wall and then perform the procedure. This way you get the support and it becomes comparatively easy to perform.

4. Repeat it for a minimum of 20 times.

The significance of the exercise

This is also a strengthening exercise for quadriceps muscle, a kind of dynamic strengthening exercise.

The most important significance of this exercise is that in addition to the quadriceps muscle, the muscle of the back of the thigh (hamstring muscle), muscle of lower leg (calf muscle and anterior shin muscle), muscle of foot is also covered.

We have already learned that quadriceps muscle brings knee straightening motion and hamstring action results in knee bending movement. So, these exercises are very important for knee joint stability.

Bullet points

1. This is a quadriceps strengthening exercises.
2. It's different from other quadriceps exercises. Having said this, movement is not isolated to one joint but multiple joint s involved.

3. Movement of all joint occurs in a closed loop.

* * *

8: Calf muscle strengthening

Strengthening of calf muscle is also as important as muscles of thigh and knee. As this muscle originates from the posterior side of knee, it's a muscle not to be ignored. However, it is very simple to perform as displayed in figure below.

Starting posture and Target posture

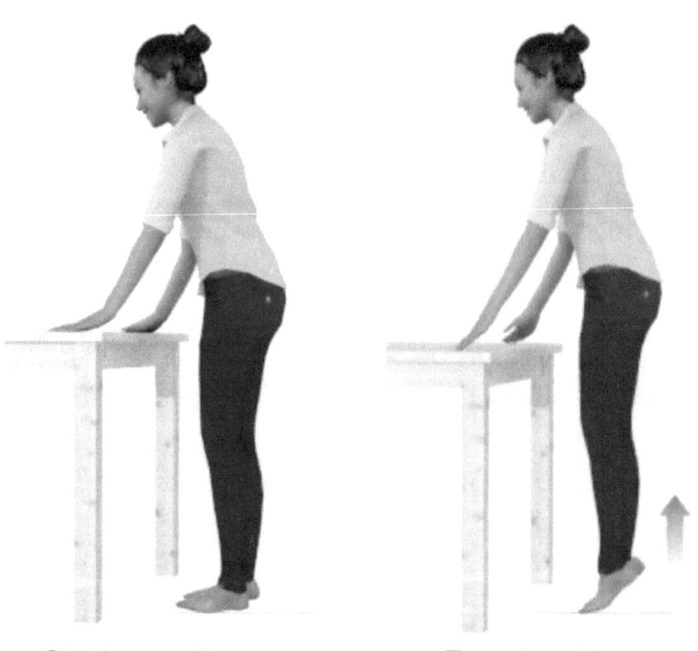

Figure 30

Description of exercise

The bulky muscle on the back of the lower leg is calf muscle and this exercise is meant for strengthening this muscle.

It is performed in a standing position and is a very easy yet very effective exercise. You may stand free without holding anything or can also take the support of the table/ plinth or any other thing for better stability or safety.

In the figure below, the model is standing by taking the support of a table. The technique explains the step-by-step method.

Technique

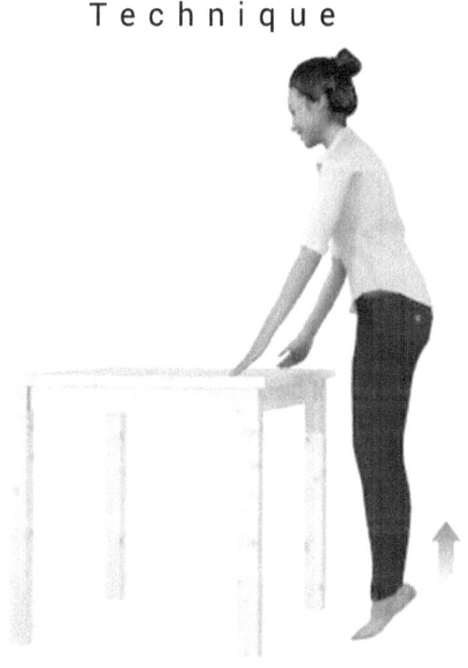

Figure 31

1. Stand straight taking the support of a table or any other things like plinth/ wall as shown in the figure.
2. You can also do these exercises without taking any support if your pain and strength allow you.
3. Now, slowly raise yourself and stand on the toes, you might feel a stretch over the calf muscle. Then lower down slowly.
4. Repeat it for a minimum of 20 times in a single session.

Significance of exercise

The calf muscle is perhaps the busiest muscle of our body and it has a very important role in standing, walking and running.

Its action causes the dorsiflexion movement (downward bending) of the foot and weakness of calf muscle greatly affects the knee biomechanics.

Calf muscle is a group of two muscle; gastrocnemius and soleus which originates from medial and lateral sides of posterior part of knee. They form the bulky part on back of lower leg and merges to form tendoachilles that inserts into calcaneum bone.

The hard tendon just below the bulky calf is tendoachilles and it is the strongest tendon of the human body.

Although there are other exercises for calf muscle, this exercise best suits the need of an OA knee sufferer.

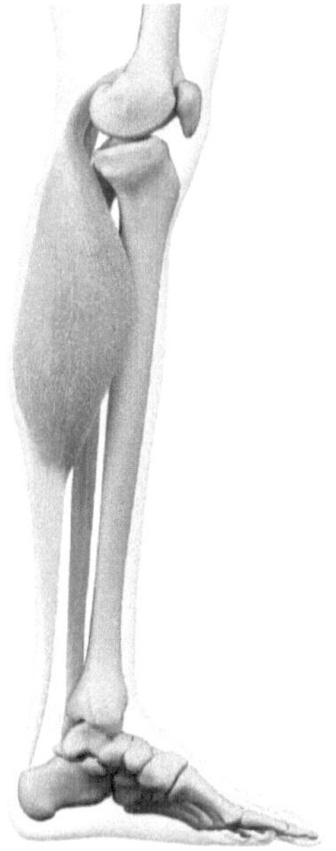

Figure 32: Calf muscle

* * *

Stretching exercise

In addition to all the factors that cause joint stiffness we discussed in the previous chapter, one of which is muscular tightness. Muscle "tightness" results from an increase in tension from active or passive mechanisms.

Passively, muscles can become shortened through postural adaptation or scarring; actively, muscles can become shorter due to spasm or contraction. Regardless of the cause, tightness limits range of motion and may create a muscle imbalance (CURRENT CONCEPTS IN MUSCLE STRETCHING FOR EXERCISE AND REHABILITATION, 2012).

Stretching is a common intervention performed during rehabilitation. Stretching is prescribed to increase muscle length and ROM, or to align collagen fibers during healing muscle and capsule.

9: Posterior knee capsule stretching exercise

In osteoarthritis knee the joint capsule on the posterior part (back) of knee commonly becomes tight and stiff. The stretching exercise is simple as displayed in the illustration.

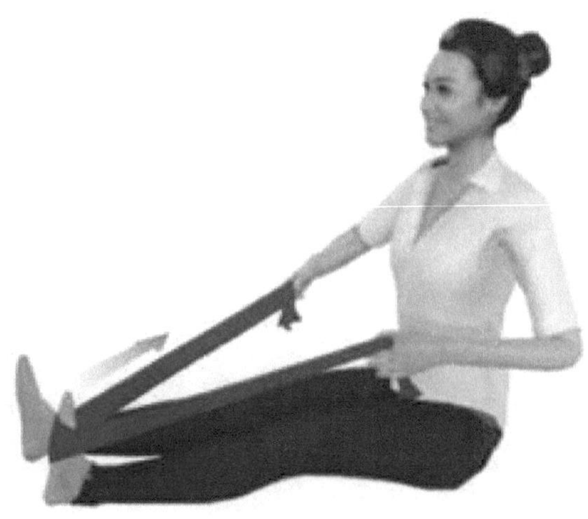

Figure 33

It is very important exercise to stretch the posterior capsule of the knee joint. For this stretching, you need a resistance band (theraband), or you may also use a towel/ bed sheet as per the availability.

Long sitting posture is the starting position; hold the resistance band as shown in the figure below. The arrow signifies the direction of pull by both of your hand. When pulling, you should allow bending of ankle joint to a point where you will fell stretch on the calf muscle.

The technique of stretching as follows.

Technique

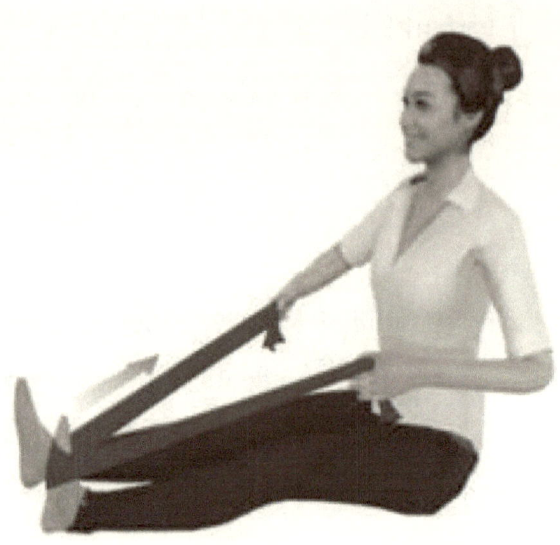

Figure 34

1. Sit in the long sitting position.

2. Take a towel or bed sheet and hold the foot with it. Grab the ends of a bedsheet with both the hand and pull it. Pull it until you feel a stretch behind the knee.

3. Pull it and hold it for 60 seconds and then release it.

4. Repeat it for 2 to 3 times in a single session.

The significance of the exercise

Like every synovial joint, knee joint space is also enclosed by a soft tissue structure called a joint capsule.

As the osteoarthritis disease process proceeds, it starts to affect the soft tissues around the articular surface. During which the posterior part of the knee joint capsule (behind the knee) is mostly affected.

This results in stiffness and contracture of the posterior capsule manifested by pain behind the knee. In my clinical practice, I have experienced that in conjunction with hot fomentation, stretching works like wonder.

Note: When you have severe pain of back of knee, then you should avoid stretching till the pain reduces. Pain can easily managed by application of pain balm over the back o knee.

10 minutes after the application of balm, apply heat treatment over the region for best result.

Bullet points:

1. The tightness of the joint capsule behind the knee is the main reason for pain on the backside of the knee.
2. This tightness also prevents to fully straighten the knee in some patients.
3. Stretching it can prove to be very beneficial to tackle both the problem.

* * *

Pain management tips

When you are regular with the exercises, there may be an occasional bout of severe acute pain. In such situation don't panic, as it's quite normal to develop during the exercises. Instead of losing hope, you must continue doing exercises.

Such pain can be managed by following simple home tips and precaution, for which you just need right information. For this, take any pain balm (ointment) and apply over the knee. Leave it for about 10 minutes.

After 10 minutes, give heat treatment over your knee. The heat treatment can be given using two methods. Use the one which best suits you.

It can be given via using:

1. Hot packs (hot water bag/hot water pads).
2. Infrared lamps.

I would recommend Infra-Red Lamp over hot pads. It has a deeper penetrating power and is more effective.

Knee braces

Why knee caps (braces) is important to use? Strengthening of muscle is important to reduce the load (offloading weight) over the knee joint. While muscle plays an important role in offloading knee joints, sometimes it may require reinforcement. This reinforcement can be provided by the use of braces.

Braces used for the knee is sometimes called a knee cap. Knee braces can be of two kinds. Each one is used in accordance with the severity of pain.

Two types of knee brace are

1. Simple knee cap.
2. Hinged knee braces.

For lesser pain, the simple knee cap is recommended. But, for more severe cases, the hinged brace is the best suit.

A hinged knee brace

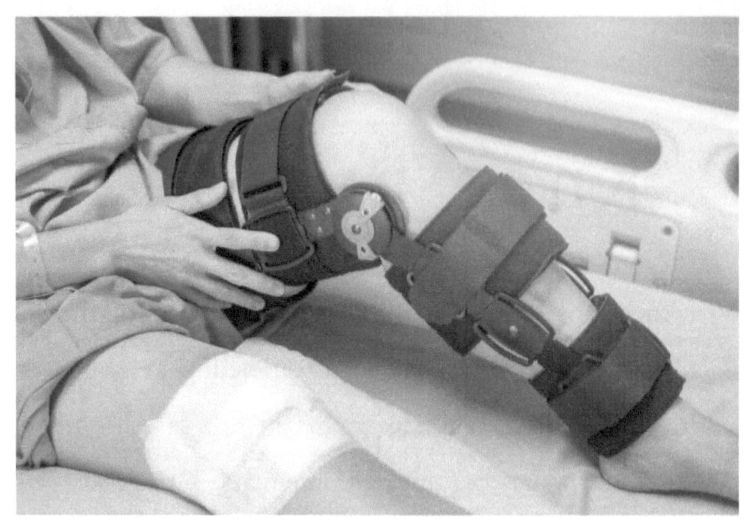

A normal knee cap

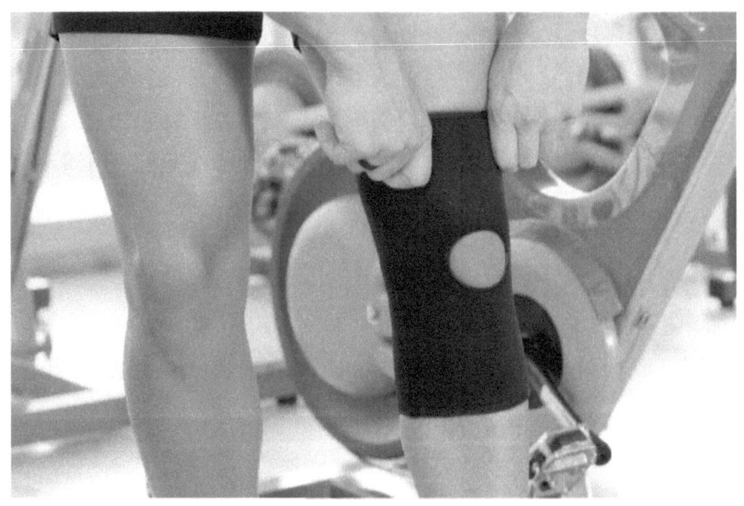

* * *

Lifestyle modification

The current treatment approach gives lifestyle modification more priority over the pharmacological treatment. Research also demonstrates that exercise(O'Reilly et al.) and lifestyle modifications can bring significant improvement in the quality of life.

The most important component of lifestyle modification includes exercises and weight management. Although exercise represents a promising lifestyle intervention, recent findings demonstrate that combining exercise and dietary weight loss is superior to implementing either intervention alone for overweight or obese individuals with knee OA(Focht).

Exercises

This whole book is focused on exercises. However, the exercises we just covered are specific to knee. Research has also revealed that aerobics, hydrotherapy, cycling and even dancing helps in the betterment of the overall life of an OA knee sufferers.

Hydrotherapy is also found to benefit osteoarthritis knee. A Brazilian study conducted on women suffering from OA knee demonstrated that a structured six-week hydrotherapy program in conjunction with an educational program led to greater improvements in pain and function in the short term when compared to an educational program alone(Dias et al.).

Recommended hydrotherapy exercises

Hydrotherapy exercises are very easy and anyone can perform it. It is performed inside the swimming pool with water level up to the waist is recommended.

Most of the land-based we discussed in this book is a part of these exercises the only difference being, it is performed inside the pool. The science behind hydrotherapy is it gives buoyancy force to the limbs that make doing the exercises easier for the knee pain sufferer.

These exercises are:

- Standing on toes.
- Walking.
- Semi-squats
- Step-up
- Single leg standing.
- Knee bending in standing.

S t a n d i n g   o n   t o e s

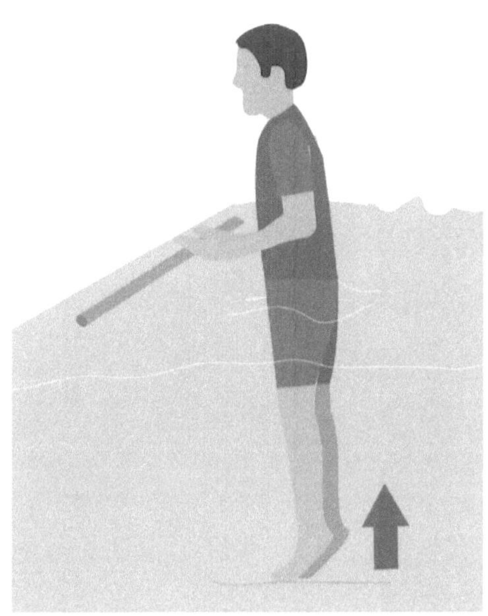

Take the support of the bar or edge of the swimming pool and stand on toes.

Semi-squat

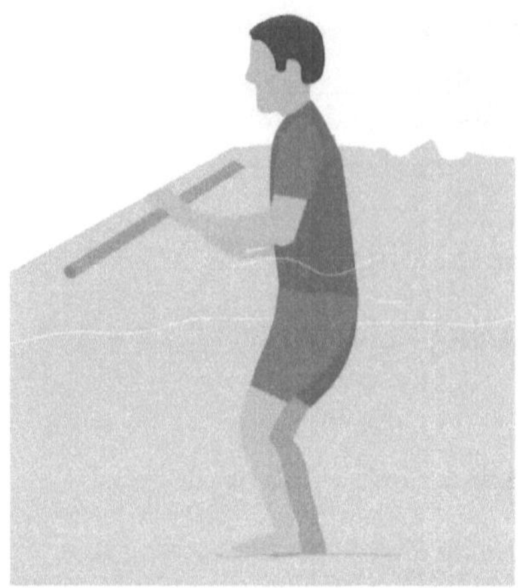

Single leg standing

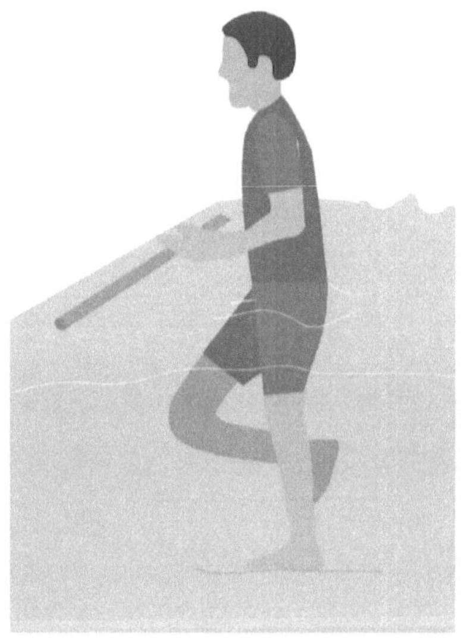

Stand on a single leg for a minimum of 10 seconds. Repeat it on the other side.

Step-up

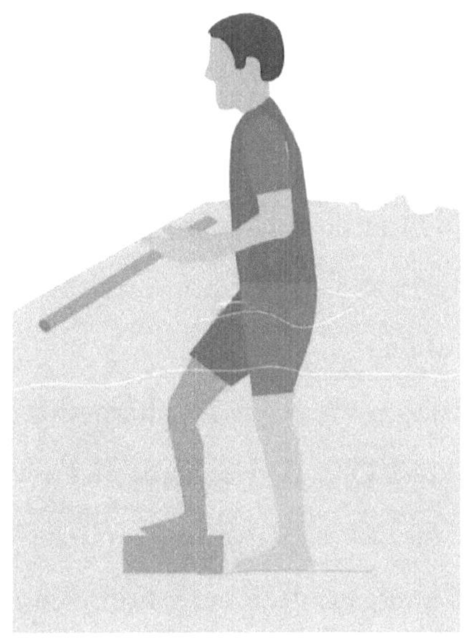

Walking

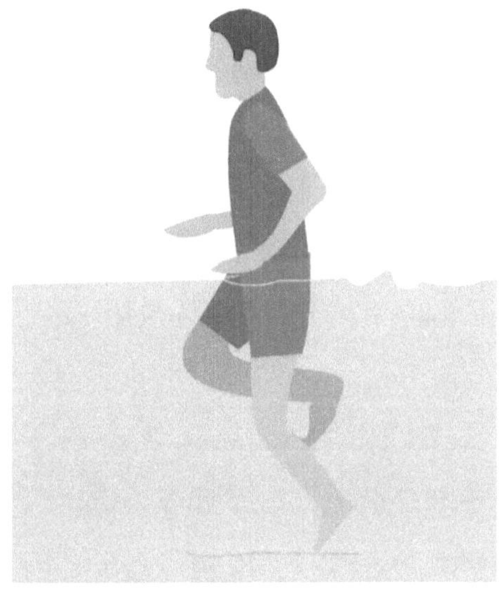

Cycling for knee pain

Lots of you might be already doing it and research(Salacinski et al.) also supports that static cycling improves the activity daily living and overall quality of life.

Cycling may be considered as an alternative exercise modality for patients with knee OA. A US study has revealed that Low-intensity cycling was as effective as high-intensity cycling in improving function and gait, decreasing pain, and increasing aerobic capacity(Mangione et al.).

Let's see some details of this research for a better understanding.

A randomized control trial was done in which 39 adults of mean age 71 years were recruited with complaints of knee pain and diagnosis of OA.

They were randomly assigned a high-intensity (70% heart rate reserve [HRR]) or low-intensity (40% HRR) exercise group for 10 weeks of stationary cycling.

Participants cycled for 25 minutes, 3 times per week. Before and after the exercise intervention they completed the Arthritis Impact Measurement Scale 2 (scale to measure the arthritis pain) for overall pain assessment

They were also assessed for the quality of these activities:

1.   Chair rise,

2.   6-minute walk test,

3.   Gait, and

4.   Graded exercise treadmill tests.

During which acute pain was reported daily with a visual analog scale and the Western Ontario and McMaster.

Result: Analysis revealed that participants in both groups significantly improved in the timed chair rise, in the 6-minute walk test, in the range of walking speeds.

Significant improvement was observed in the amount of overall pain relief, and in aerobic capacity. No differences between groups were found. Daily pain reports suggested that cycling did not increase acute pain in either group.

Why should osteoarthritis patients lose weight?

An obese person with knee OA had a greater risk of progression of structural change in the knee and a greater risk of developing OA in the knee.

Significant relationships between even small increases in body mass index and prevalence of knee OA have been consistently documented. Findings from the Framingham Heart study and the first National Health and Nutrition Examination Survey (NHANES I) demonstrated that individuals with the highest body weights had the greatest risk of developing knee OA. Prospective studies also revealed that individuals who become overweight or obese have a significantly greater risk of developing knee OA and that successful weight loss substantially reduces the risk of knee OA(Focht).

Activity restriction for OA knee sufferer

There are certain activities that can potentially accelerate the degenerative process of OA knee. It is recommend to avoid such activities.

These activities are

1. Squatting.
2. Crossed leg sitting.
3. Stair climbing.

* * *

Late stage OA knee

The late stage is a serious stage that severely affects the mobility of sufferers and even they may become bed rid. Knee looks swollen and standing walking becomes a struggle. The severity at this stage is clearly visible in the X-ray radiograph.

The joint space between bones is dramatically reduced—the articular surface becomes rough and cartilage is almost completely gone. The synovial fluid is decreased dramatically, and it no longer helps reduce the friction among the moving parts of a joint.

In such cases, knee replacement surgery is recommended. I have seen a significant change in the lives of people with replacement surgery.

There are two kinds of replacement surgery, a total knee replacement (TKR), and partial knee replacement (PKR). Your surgeon will make the decision about the surgical procedure that better solves the purpose depending upon the level of articular degradation. Though, research reveals that PKR is as effective TKR and is also cost-effective(David).

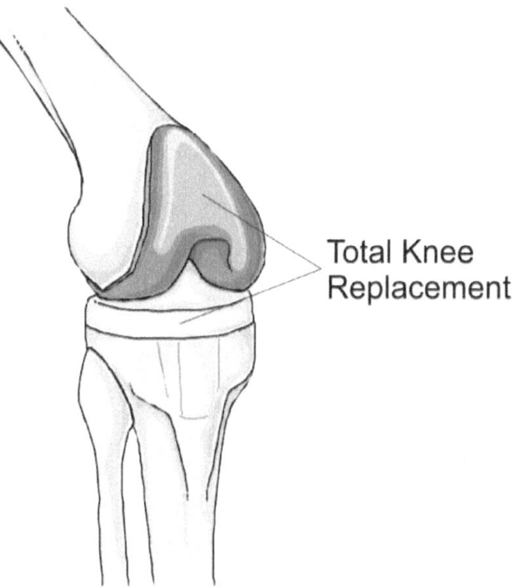

Figure 35: Total Knee Replacement

How exercises can help at this stage?

The purpose of exercises in this stage is to make the knee joint ready for surgery. Optimum muscle strength is required preoperatively to prevent secondary complications after the surgery.

It affects how soon and better you recover from the surgery. The most important post-surgical complication is disuse muscle atrophy which affects the gait (walking pattern). Exercises prevent this complication; also exercises improve blood circulation around the knee which is important for recovery from surgery.

Exercises in late stage

Except for the land-based exercises you can perform all the exercises we have discussed above.

Let me once again mention those exercises, for more details on exercises you may refer back to the respective chapters.

1. Static quadriceps exercise.

2. Dynamic quadriceps exercise.

3. Adductor strengthening exercise.

4.	Abductor strengthening exercise.

5.	Short abductor strengthening exercise.

95

After the surgery, the exercise is started right form the next day post-surgery. There is a set of exercise that you need to perform after replacement surgery and it is called a postoperative exercise protocol.

This protocol is very important for minimizing the complications, promotes healing and has an impact on your walking pattern. The postoperative protocol is beyond the scope of this book.

* * *

Final word

OA knee pain can be frustrating; sometimes it may seem that nothing is working.

But, a perfect combination of home exercise, your physiotherapist's help, the use of proper braces and lifestyle modification can have an immense effect on your pain-free lifestyle.

With these words, I conclude my book on knee pain. I hope you find it worth and it would be my success if it helps you relieve your pain.

Happy healing!

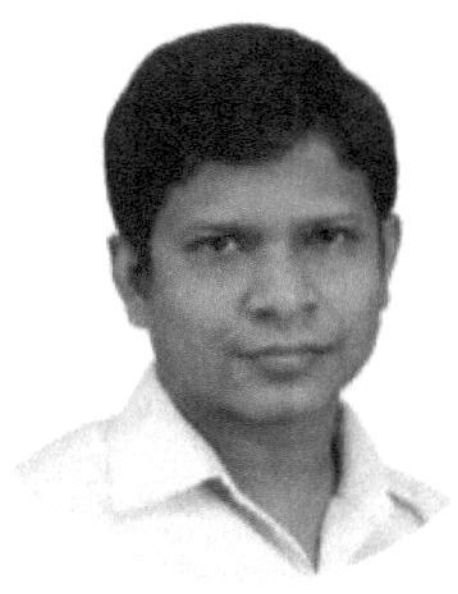

About the author

The author is a physiotherapist practicing for the last 11 years. He owns a successful physiotherapy center named "Physiofirst" at Rourkela, Odisha, India.

He holds a Bachelor's in Physiotherapy (BPT) from SVNIRTAR (Swami Vivekananda National Institute of rehabilitation and research), one of the prestigious physiotherapy schools of India.

You can find many other useful resources in his blog *www.physiosunit.com*, His knowledge and invaluable experience in the field is proving beneficial to many.

Email him: sunitekka@gmail.com

Blog: www.physiosunit.com

Join him: www.facebook.com/physiocapsule

Other titles from the author

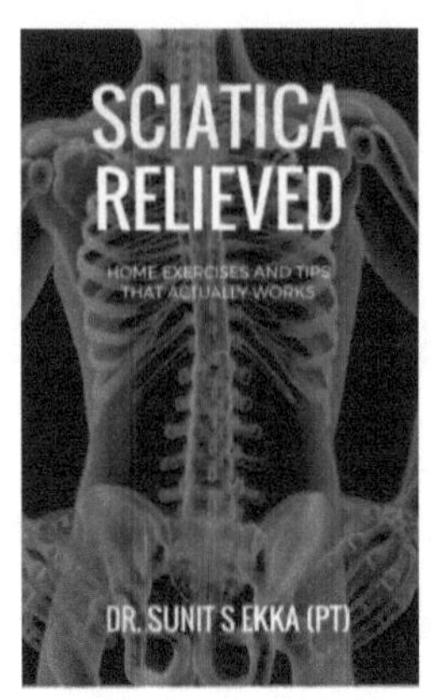

Sciatica Relieved:

Home Exercises and Tips That Actually Works

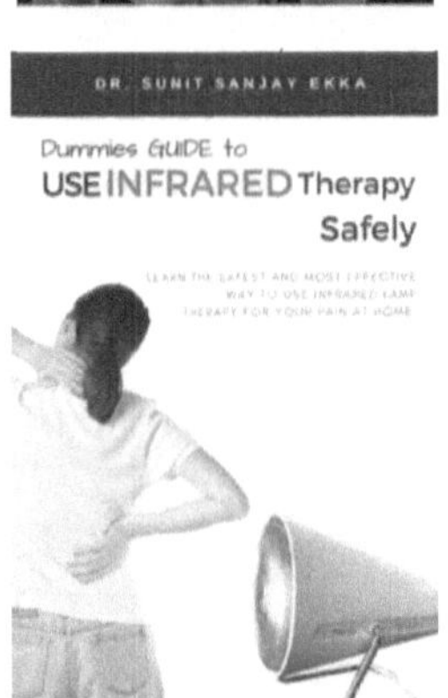

Dummies Guide to Use Infrared Therapy safely:

Learn the safest and most effective way to use infrared therapy for your pain at home

R e f e r e n c e s :

Charlesworth, Jonathon, et al. "Osteoarthritis- a Systematic Review of Long-Term Safety Implications for Osteoarthritis of the Knee." *BMC Musculoskeletal Disorders*, vol. 20, no. 1, Apr. 2019, p. 151, doi:10.1186/s12891-019-2525-0.

David, J. Beard. *The Clinical and Cost-Effectiveness of Total versus Partial Knee Replacement in Patients with Medial Compartment Osteoarthritis (TOPKAT): 5-Year Outcomes of a Randomised Controlled Trial - The Lancet.* https://www.thelancet.com/journals/lancet/article/PIIS0140-6736(19)31281-4/fulltext. Accessed 22 Oct. 2019.

Dias, João Marcos, et al. "Hydrotherapy Improves Pain and Function in Older Women with Knee Osteoarthritis: A Randomized Controlled Trial." *Brazilian Journal of Physical Therapy*, vol. 21, no. 6, 2017, pp. 449–56, doi:10.1016/j.bjpt.2017.06.012. PubMed, 28733093.

Focht, Brian C. "Move to Improve: How Knee Osteoarthritis Patients Can Use Exercise to Enhance Quality of Life." *ACSM's Health & Fitness Journal*, vol. 16, no. 5, Sept. 2012, pp. 24–28, doi:10.1249/FIT0b013e318264cae8. PubMed, 23359219.

Fransen, Marlene, et al. "Exercise for Osteoarthritis of the Knee: A Cochrane Systematic Review." *British Journal of Sports Medicine*, vol. 49, no. 24, Dec. 2015, p. 1554, doi:10.1136/bjsports-2015-095424.

Heidari, Behzad. "Knee Osteoarthritis Prevalence, Risk Factors, Pathogenesis and Features: Part I." *Caspian Journal of Internal Medicine*, vol. 2, no. 2, 2011, pp. 205–12. PubMed, 24024017.

KELLGREN, J. H., and J. S. LAWRENCE. "Radiological Assessment of Osteo-Arthrosis." *Annals of the Rheumatic Diseases*, vol. 16, no. 4, Dec. 1957, pp. 494–502, doi:10.1136/ard.16.4.494. PubMed, 13498604.

Khoja, Samannaaz S., et al. "Recommendation Rates for Physical Therapy, Lifestyle Counseling and Pain Medications for Managing Knee Osteoarthritis in Ambulatory Care Settings. Cross-Sectional Analysis of the National Ambulatory Care Survey (2007-2015)." *Arthritis Care & Research*, vol. 0, no. ja, Oct. 2019, doi:10.1002/acr.24064.

Kohn, Mark D., et al. "Classifications in Brief: Kellgren-Lawrence Classification of Osteoarthritis." *Clinical Orthopaedics and Related Research*, vol. 474, no. 8, Aug. 2016, pp. 1886–93, doi:10.1007/s11999-016-4732-4. PubMed, 26872913.

Lespasio, Michelle J., et al. "Knee Osteoarthritis: A Primer." *The Permanente Journal*, vol. 21, 2017, pp. 16–183, doi:10.7812/TPP/16-183. PubMed, 29035179.

Mangione, Kathleen, et al. "The Effects of High-Intensity and Low-Intensity Cycle Ergometry in Older Adults With Knee Osteoarthritis." *The Journals of Gerontology. Series A, Biological Sciences and Medical Sciences*, vol. 54, May 1999, pp. M184-90, doi:10.1093/gerona/54.4.M184.

O'Reilly, Sheila C., et al. "Effectiveness of Home Exercise on Pain and Disability from Osteoarthritis of the Knee: A Randomised Controlled Trial." *Annals of the Rheumatic Diseases*, vol. 58, no. 1, Jan. 1999, p. 15, doi:10.1136/ard.58.1.15.

Salacinski, Amanda J., et al. "The Effects of Group Cycling on Gait and Pain-Related Disability in Individuals With Mild-to-Moderate Knee Osteoarthritis: A Randomized Controlled Trial." *Journal of Orthopaedic & Sports Physical Therapy*, vol. 42, no. 12, Dec. 2012, pp. 985–95, doi:10.2519/jospt.2012.3813.

Slemenda, Charles, et al. "Quadriceps Weakness and Osteoarthritis of the Knee." *Annals of Internal Medicine*, vol. 127, no. 2, July 1997, pp. 97–104, doi:10.7326/0003-4819-127-2-199707150-00001.

Kevin R. Vincent, H. K. (2012). Resistance Exercise for Knee Osteoarthritis. *PM & R : the journal of injury, function, and rehabilitation* , vol. 4,5 Suppl.